Nurse-led Primary Care

Learning from PMS pilots

Richard Lewis

Foreword by the Chief Nursing Officer

King's **Fund**

Published by
King's Fund Publishing
11–13 Cavendish Square
London W1G 0AN

© King's Fund 2001

First published 2001

ISBN 1 85717 447 X

A CIP catalogue record for this book is available from the British Library

Available from:
King's Fund Bookshop
11–13 Cavendish Square
LONDON
W1G 0AN

Tel: 020 7307 2591
Fax: 020 7307 2801

Printed and bound in Great Britain

Cover illustration: creativ collection

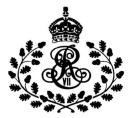

Contents

Acknowledgements

I would like to thank the following from the nurse-led pilot sites who generously gave their time to this evaluation:

Catherine Baraniak

Kate Cernik

Lance Gardner

Sarah Healey

Alison Holbourne

Norma House

Maggie Ioagnou

Wendy Johnson

Teresa Kearney

Carol Latham

Mary Mathias

Barbara Rennells

Patricia Robinson

James Savage

Barbara Stuttle

I am also grateful to Steve Gillam, Pippa Gough, Frances Pickersgill and Rebecca Rosen for their valuable comments on early drafts of the report.

Foreword

The development of personal medical services (PMS) pilots in primary care has been an opportunity to do things differently. The pilots have provided a new way of working and new opportunities for GPs to pursue a different career path, as well as meeting different, locally relevant objectives.

All the PMS pilots have also provided opportunities for nurses to work in new ways. Whether working in a team with salaried GPs, or providing specialist services for vulnerable populations, nurses have been an essential element of the whole PMS picture. But there is a small group of nurses who have contributed to PMS pilots in a very particular way. These are nurses who have personally led the new services, taking on the professional and managerial burden of creating the pilot's objectives, building the multi-professional team, managing the expenditure, and ensuring that the ultimate beneficiaries of this radical and sometimes challenging change are patients and service users.

This report explores the experiences of nine of these pioneer nurses. Against a background of the development of PMS and the evolution of nursing roles in primary care, the report analyses data collected through two focus groups of nurse leads. The nature and characteristics of nurse-led pilots are described and the nurses explore their value systems, their model of care, and their relationships with other professionals and with hospital services.

It is never easy to be first, and it is not easy to expose your anxieties, frustrations and less-than-ideal experiences to the scrutiny of others. But there is a great deal to be learned from this thoughtful, realistic and ultimately optimistic appraisal of the early years of these nurse-led pilots.

I am grateful to them for their courage, their honesty and their leadership. I hope that this report encourages all of us to be more supportive and responsive to the leaders and pioneers amongst us. I also hope that it encourages many more nurses to grasp opportunities that are offered to 'do things differently' to improve services for patients.

Sarah Mullally
Chief Nursing Officer
London, March 2001

Executive summary

In 1998, the Secretary of State approved nine PMS pilots to offer 'nurse-led' primary care. These pilots were designed to maximise the use of nursing skills and to allow nurses to exercise leadership within the primary health care team. This report describes the experiences of the nine nurse leads as they have developed their pilots.

Government policy has emphasised the need to examine the mix of skills within the NHS, in particular to break down existing demarcations between medical and nursing roles. The Chief Nursing Officer has identified ten key roles that all nurses with appropriate skills might undertake. In primary care, the role and number of nurses has increased substantially during the 1990s. Much attention has been placed on the role of the nurse practitioner. There is a growing body of research evidence which suggests that these nurses can offer care that is similar in quality and cost to that of doctors in a number of settings. Nurse-led PMS pilots have begun to put into practice a new model of care that is consistent with the Government's objectives for the NHS.

The pilots

Nine nurse-led sites 'went live' in the first wave of PMS pilots. Five pilots were managed by community NHS trusts, two pilots were managed by existing GP practices and two pilots were managed by nurses acting as independent contractors. In the latter two practices, nurses acted as the employers of other team members, including GPs.

Pilots shared a number of priorities, including: serving vulnerable populations (such as refugees or homeless people); providing patient-focused care; breaking down professional boundaries; improving access to services; community development and/or patient empowerment; and developing partnerships with other agencies and community groups. The nine pilots are serving very different numbers of patients. In some pilots, the list of registered patients is very small. In general, nurse-led pilots have relatively large primary health care teams when compared to the average for general practice.

What is nurse-led care?

Nurse leads define 'nurse-led' care as the combination of extended nursing roles and a culture that promotes equality between different professions and the empowerment of patients. Because of the emphasis on vulnerable populations, nurse leads perceive that local 'traditional' general practices are directing particular patients to the pilots rather than providing services themselves.

Pushing back the professional boundaries

Nurse leads were concerned that the number of nurse practitioners in primary care (including NHS Direct) was growing without sufficient attention nationally on establishing agreed competencies, standards or training. At local level, clinical governance processes had not led to any quality assurance in relation to the work of the nine pilots.

Within their own pilots, nurse leads have mostly been successful in establishing a new model for interprofessional working. However, in one pilot significant disagreements over the respective roles of nurses and doctors had caused two successive nurse leads to leave the team. Nurse leads had experienced some hostility to their pilots from other local doctors. Nurse leads perceived that this hostility was greatest if they attempted to offer services to a mainstream population, rather than to disadvantaged groups.

Nurse leads have generally been successful in negotiating the right to access diagnostic services directly and to make and receive referrals from the hospital sector. However, this has mostly relied on informal arrangements and few nurse leads have agreements with all hospital specialties. Some consultants still insist on communicating only with the pilot doctor.

Pilot implementation

Nurse leads have been presented with a number of obstacles in implementing their pilots. Nurses are not eligible to sign benefits or death certificates, or to officially register patients (this must be formally done by a GP). In addition, the ability of nurses to prescribe is (currently) highly restricted.

Nurse leads employed by community NHS trusts identified a lack of autonomy and, in some cases, support in developing their pilots. NHS trusts have proved bureaucratic and not sufficiently responsive to the day-to-day needs of a primary care team. However, independent contractor nurse leads, while autonomous, have suffered from isolation. The existence of 'local champions' has been important in the success of the pilots.

Conclusions

More than two years into their pilots, the nine nurse leads have achieved a great deal and are putting into place the Government's radical vision for health care. There are a number of lessons to be learnt:

- 'Nurse-led' care is not simply a description of the role of nurses but describes also a culture of professional equality and patient-focused services.

- This new model of care has created come local controversy and, in particular, hostility from doctors. Nurse leadership is but a further change heralded by PMS pilots that have, more generally, raised the hackles of a section of 'traditional' general practice. Nevertheless, the pilots have managed to negotiate a new doctor–nurse relationship within primary care and with hospital colleagues.

- Nurse-led pilots have tended to serve vulnerable populations, often poorly served by general practice. They have proved popular with these patients, although this raises interesting ethical issues. Traditional general practices are perceived now to direct patients to the nurse-led pilots, raising the spectre of a two-tier service –

with the disadvantaged receiving their care from nurses and the mainstream population from doctors.

- Current NHS and welfare regulation are not sufficiently sensitive to the new role of nurses and need review (in the case of nurse prescribing, changes are imminent). Community NHS trust-managed schemes are likely to transfer to primary care trusts (PCTs) when these have been established. It is far from clear whether this will resolve the problems of bureaucracy that beset community trust pilots. Nor is it clear whether medically dominated PCTs will support the nurse-led model.

- A new infrastructure is required to support new nursing roles. In particular, more clarity is required over the competencies, training and quality assurance of nurse practitioner services. Nurse leads perceived that they had received little in the way of support from their professional bodies.

The nurse-led pilots have begun to implement the Government's strategy for nursing. Emerging research suggests that this model of care is popular with patients (although evidence on the cost-effectiveness of nurse-led pilots is not available). However, it is not clear whether there are sufficient nurses available and willing to follow the example set by the nine nurse leads.

1. Introduction

This report considers two key aspects of Government health policy: the introduction of personal medical services (PMS) pilots as a means to increase the responsiveness and effectiveness of primary care; and the renegotiation of the respective roles of professionals within the primary health care team, specifically enhancing the contribution to care made by nurses. These two policy streams have come together in the advent of 'nurse-led' PMS pilots – a small, but important, group of primary health care teams that are led by nurses, and that have the development of nursing roles as a key objective.

In announcing a first wave of PMS pilots, Frank Dobson, then Secretary of State for Health, specifically encouraged nurses to use them as an opportunity to develop a new kind of primary care: a primary care that maximised the nursing contribution as well as the leadership qualities of nurses themselves. Subsequently, nine nurse-led pilots were approved to begin operation on 1 April 1998. These nine initiatives provide the focus for this report: what sort of primary care have they developed; what has been their experience of 'nurse leadership' so far; and what might we learn about the implementation of the Government's policy to extend nursing roles?

Personal medical services pilots

PMS pilots, introduced following the 1997 NHS (Primary Care) Act, marked an important departure in the policies of successive governments towards primary care. Primary care has been (and largely still is) focused on the work of GPs. Prior to the Act, all GP principals held individual contracts with the Secretary of State for Health, were independent contractors and were responsible for the direct employment of practice staff, including practice nurses and a range of other practice-based professionals. The relationship between GPs and the NHS was largely governed through collective bargaining between the General Practice Committee (formerly the General Medical Services Committee) of the British Medical Association and the

Department of Health. The result was a national general medical services (GMS) contract. Local involvement in, and discretion over, the activities of GPs was limited.

PMS pilots introduced some significant changes to the *status quo*:

- Contracts (and budgets) were drawn up and negotiated locally between the health authority (or, later, the primary care trust) and the primary care provider.
- New types of provider were able to contract to provide primary medical services. These included community NHS trusts, independent nurses and, exceptionally, limited companies.
- New opportunities for the salaried employment of GPs were created, offering an alternative to the independent contractor model.

While the first wave of pilots was modest in size, with 83 pilots going 'live' in April 1998, numbers soon grew rapidly.[1] By the third wave in 2001, the Government estimated that 20 per cent of GPs would be covered by PMS contracts.

PMS pilots are significant for primary care nursing. They are already introducing new roles and responsibilities for nurses,[2] and significant developmental resources are being made to encourage the employment of a new cadre of 'nurse practitioners'. In particular, pilots that are currently managed by NHS trusts and that may, in the future, transfer to PCTs, are introducing new power structures within primary health care teams. Through the salaried employment of the whole team, the employer–employee dimension that has so long characterised the GP–nurse relationship is removed. Exceptionally, independent contractor nurses are employing the other members of the team. These new organisational forms open up new possibilities for interprofessional relations.

The challenge for nursing

In March 2000, the Government announced a significant increase in the resources available to the NHS. These resources were not simply a 'one-off' bonanza, but were part of a five-year plan that would increase spending, in real terms, by 35 per cent.

However, this Government largesse came with strings attached. If the Government was going to heed the continuing cries for more money that emanated from within the NHS, it would expect wholesale changes in the way in which the NHS was to operate in return.[3]

At the time of his announcement, Tony Blair set the NHS five key challenges that formed a new 'deal' between government and the health service. One challenge was to 'strip out unnecessary demarcations, introduce more flexible training and working practices, and ensure that doctors do not use time dealing with patients who could be treated safely by other health care staff'. Health Secretary Alan Milburn, in his address to the Annual Congress of the Royal College of Nursing, stressed that nurses were at the centre of the Government's plans for modernisation and promised 'a health service which liberates nurses not limits them'. Nurses were, he suggested, the new leaders of change, and nursing values were at one with the values that he wanted to underpin the NHS: care, compassion, professionalism and dedication.[4]

The Secretary of State identified ten nurse roles that should, in the future, become widespread throughout the NHS (later described as the Chief Nursing Officer's 'ten key roles for nurses' – see Box 1.1). These roles built on the experience and achievements of leaders in the field; if opportunities to fulfil these roles were available to some then they should be available to all appropriately skilled nurses. Nurses of the future look set to move into territory hitherto firmly occupied by doctors.

This theme of shuffling the professional pack was one that was embellished in the *NHS Plan*. This set out a challenging agenda for the NHS. The post-Plan NHS was to be responsive, convenient and tailored to individual needs. Access to primary and intermediate care services was particularly highlighted. Nurses were to act as linchpins of this new NHS. According to the Government, 'pressure on GP services will be eased as nurses and other community staff … take on more tasks.'[5] Instant access to primary care advice via NHS Direct, rapid access within the GP surgery, the encouragement of GPs to develop sub-specialisms all rely on nurses carrying out extended roles. A similar agenda is unfolding for hospital and community nursing, with more than 1000 nurse consultants promised, together with the re-invention of the hospital matron.

Box 1.1: Chief Nursing Officer's ten key roles for nurses

1. Order diagnostic investigations (e.g. pathology tests and x-rays).
2. Make and receive referrals direct (e.g. to a therapist or pain consultant).
3. Admit and discharge patients for specified conditions and within agreed protocols.
4. Manage patient caseloads (e.g. for diabetes and rheumatology).
5. Run clinics (e.g. ophthalmology or dermatology).
6. Prescribe medicines and treatment.
7. Carry out a wide range of resuscitation procedures, including defibrillation.
8. Perform minor surgery and out-patient procedures.
9. Triage patients using the latest IT to the most appropriate health professional.
10. Take a lead in the way local health services are organised and in the way they are run.

The evolving role of the primary care nurse

The 1990s saw a rapid increase in the employment of practice nursing. Between 1989 and 1999, the number of whole time equivalent practice nurses in England more than doubled from 4632 to 10,689.[6] Practice nurses were seen as an increasingly essential component of the primary health care team, not least because the re-structured GMS GP contract included financial incentives that encouraged the provision of a wide range of services that were particularly suited to nurses.

A key debate within primary care has concerned the appropriate skill-mix in relation to medical and nursing roles. Increasingly, governments have seen substitution between nurses and doctors as a policy response to the apparent shortage of GPs. Much of this attention has focused on the role of the 'nurse practitioner'. This is a slippery term; nurse practitioner status is not formally recognised by the United Kingdom Central Council (UKCC), the body that currently regulates the nursing profession. However, the Royal College of Nursing has provided a role definition that covers the work of nurse practitioners within a primary care setting. In its view, the nurse practitioner is:

An advanced level clinical nurse who through extra education and training is able to practice autonomously, making clinical decisions and instigating treatment decisions based on those decisions, and is fully accountable for her own practice.[7]

The ability of nurse practitioners to substitute effectively for doctors in a wide range of settings is now well demonstrated both in the United States and in the UK. Randomised controlled trials have provided ample evidence to suggest that care by nurse practitioners is similar in quality and cost to that provided by doctors. In addition, patient satisfaction with nurse practitioner care is comparable, if not higher, than that resulting from care provided by a doctor.[8,9,10,11] A Department of Health-sponsored evaluation also suggested that nurse practitioners were able to provide services that are acceptable to patients and (where data were available) at similar or lower cost than that of doctors.[12]

The ability of nurses to prescribe a limited range of products has been tentatively introduced.[13] However, a fundamental review of non-medical prescribing has been undertaken and proposals are currently under consultation.[14] It is proposed that, following suitable training, independent prescribing rights are held by those nurses holding a specialist practitioner qualification recognised on the UKCC professional register or a clinically based qualification, such as a nurse practitioner degree.[15]

Yet finding an appropriate new equilibrium between medical and nursing roles has not been without its difficulties and tensions. Certainly, both doctors and nurses acknowledge that the boundaries between them are blurring. For doctors, this has been something to fear. For nurses, there is frustration in the perceived subservience of their role in relation to that of doctors. Very often, medical colleagues also act as primary care nurses' employers, emphasising the unequal relationship that exists.[16] Interprofessional collaboration may require equal status and power if it is to be effective.[17] As two commentators have caricatured interprofessional relations:

Nurses, more assertive, educated, and competent than ever before, resent what they see as continuing put downs by a profession holding all the cards. Doctors, puzzled and unaccustomed to being challenged, are themselves resentful at the apparent undervaluing of their competence, knowledge, and skills by nurses, the public, and policymakers. Everyone is confused.[18]

So, are doctors and nurses simply two tribes with different world-views, using the patient as their battleground? A study of medical and nursing cultures suggested that, in fact, there are no distinguishable differences between the 'core values' that underpin both professions. However, their different cultures and histories lead to alternative interpretations as to how these values might be pursued in practice. Tensions are also evident *within* the nursing profession as changes in skill-mix shift roles between different branches of primary care nursing. One consequence of changing skill-mix and care substitution is a decline in professional identities. This may be necessary if entrenched behaviours are to change. Nevertheless, a strong professional identity is associated with good teamwork and morale, and a loss of identity may result in reduced quality of care.[19]

Nurse-led PMS pilots appear to invert the common, medically dominated culture of primary care and to radically restructure professional identity. One PMS pilot nurse lead has suggested that formal professional titles act as a barrier to teamwork and that nurse-led pilots should introduce 'democratically organised teams with decision-making based on consensus'. As a consequence, greater emphasis should be placed on the particular skills and expertise of each individual team member.[20] Has this blurring of professional identities led to reduced morale? An evaluation of this pilot suggests the opposite. Despite initial scepticism and even anger, staff within this practice soon expressed great enthusiasm.[21]

PMS pilots already appear to be in the vanguard of change in relation to skill-mix, whether or not they are formally nurse led. Nurse roles are evolving rapidly in practice-based pilots and new nurse roles are being developed, such as triage and nurse-led chronic disease management.[22,23]

How have patients adapted to these changes in practice? An evaluation of patient perceptions of nurse-led care suggests that they have found the new model acceptable. Indeed, many patients expressed a preference to see the nurse rather than the doctor.

Patients valued the nurse-led service because it offered continuity and stability, was accessible and personalised, and because the nurse took an interest in people's material and domestic situations. Interestingly, in this evaluation these were the same attributes that patients associated with the previous, much-valued GP care that they had received prior to the pilot's inception.[24] This poses a question – is successful nurse-led care simply the same as 'good' primary medical care?

Evaluation methods

This evaluation focuses on the views and perceptions of the pilot nurse leads themselves. Therefore, the nine nurses (and in some cases their immediate managers, where they have been heavily involved in establishing the pilots) have provided the data upon which this report is based. Clearly, others who have been involved in the pilots (whether as commissioners, neighbouring practices or as patients) may have a very different view of events. These other perspectives are important but have not been the subject of this research.

The main form of data collection has been through two focus groups (held in June and December 2000). Seven of the nine sites attended the first focus group and four sites were represented at the second. The focus groups were intended to allow the participants to explore their experiences and to distil lessons that might be important for other nurses following in their footsteps and, indeed, for the wider NHS in considering the role of nurses within primary care.

Prior to the first focus group, all sites were sent a questionnaire. This was designed to collect basic information about each pilot, as well as the qualitative views of the nurse leads about the perceived success of the pilots in meeting their objectives and any lessons learnt through implementation. Questionnaires were completed by all pilots. Subsequently, the questionnaire was extended to collect data systematically about the relationship with the acute hospital sector (a topic that emerged as significant during the first focus group and which is discussed in this report).

This evaluation of nurse-led pilots has also drawn upon the larger scale evaluation of first wave PMS pilots being carried out by the King's Fund (in association with the

National Primary Care Research and Development Centre). This evaluation has used a range of qualitative and quantitative methods, and incorporated two of the nine nurse-led sites.[25]

Conclusion

Nurse-led PMS pilots are the latest thrust of an evolving policy to enhance the contribution that nurses make to primary care. No doubt, different protagonists have different motivations for this. Government may see nurse-led care as a means to avoid a GP recruitment crisis; nurses may see it as an opportunity to establish autonomous practice. It has been noted that, unlike doctors, nurses find their professional futures shaped predominantly by external factors, whether these be doctors as employers, the economics of care or changes to the health system generally.[26] Nurse-led PMS pilots appear to offer nurses an opportunity to shape their professional development themselves.

However, notwithstanding the advances already made by PMS pilots, nurse-led pilots face obstacles that reflect the medically dominated history of NHS administration. These include severe limitations on nurses' ability to prescribe autonomously, their inability to register patients directly and restrictions on their powers of certification, for example in the case of death or mental health section.[27] This degree of restriction on autonomous practice contrasts with the United States, where nurse practitioners practice without any requirement for physician supervision or collaboration in 50 per cent of states. In addition, nurse practitioners in all states are directly reimbursed for services under Medicaid (the government health programme for the poor).[28]

The Government's proposals for enhanced roles for nursing are supported by a raft of evidence about the effectiveness of nursing care in different settings. Yet how, and whether, these roles can be effectively translated into the mainstream of primary care is a rather different question. In this respect, much of the Government's thinking appears to be relatively untested. As they reach the end of their third year of operation, this report seeks to describe and examine the experiences of the first nine nurse-led pilots. These nurses are the trail-blazers for the new cadre of nurses upon which the NHS Plan relies.

2. The nine nurse-led pilots

Brief details of the nine nurse-led PMS pilot sites are presented in Table 2.1.

Pilot characteristics

Eight of the nine pilots were newly established practices, providing services where none had before been provided. In one case, the nurse-led pilot was awarded a vacant list following the death of the incumbent GP. Six of the nine pilots were designed to provide services to specifically targeted populations (although, not necessarily exclusively to these populations) or to increase access to primary care for the general population in 'under-doctored' areas. The most common population groups targeted were those of homeless people (five pilots) and refugees and asylum seekers (two pilots).

While the 'official' start date of first wave PMS pilots was intended to be 1 April 1998, only two pilots were operational at that time. Several pilots experienced considerable delays as they prepared themselves to provide services. This was due to the need to recruit team members or to secure premises. The majority of pilots were operational within six months of the intended start date. One pilot became operational in December 1999, more than a year and a half after the intended starting date.

Contracts, organisation and management

The nine pilots adopted one of three organisational and contractual approaches. The most common arrangement was for the pilot to be managed by a community NHS trust that held a contract with the local health authority (five pilots). Two pilots were managed by existing general practices that established branch surgeries or quasi-independent organisations. In one case, the contract holder was a PMS practice and, in the other, a GMS practice. Finally, two pilots were provided by independently contracted nurses who contracted on their own behalf with their local health authority and directly employed practice staff.

Four of the nine pilots contracted to provide PMS 'Plus' services (i.e. services that are beyond those provided as standard within a general practice). In three of these pilots, the 'Plus' element comprised community nursing services; in the other, child development and midwifery services.

Pilot objectives

Pilots were established with a wide range of individual objectives. However, a number of themes emerged across pilots. These included:

- serving vulnerable populations (five pilots)
- providing 'patient-focused' or 'user-friendly' services (four pilots)
- developing the clinical skills of team members and/or breaking down professional boundaries (four pilots)
- improving patient access to primary care (four pilots)
- community development and/or patient empowerment (four pilots)
- developing partnerships with other agencies, voluntary or community groups (two pilots).

List size and team composition

By December 2000 (two years and eight months after their intended start dates), the nine pilots displayed a wide range in the number of registered patients. List sizes ranged from 500 to 2600 patients, with a mean average of 1311 patients. Some of the pilots with particularly low list sizes were serving well-defined populations with particularly high needs (for example, pilots serving exclusively homeless populations). In other cases, pilots had experienced a rapid on-take of patients since their establishment and were serving populations of 2000 or more.

The composition of the clinical teams also varies widely among pilots. There is no clear pattern between list size and size of the clinical team. For example, the Appleton Primary Care Pilot and the Valley Park Surgery are both serving 1000 patients but have significantly different clinical teams. In some cases, the ratio of clinicians to patients might be considered quite high compared to 'traditional' general practice. An 'average' GP principal is likely to have a registered list of 1845 patients (or 1965 per whole time equivalent GP). Each principal will, on average, work with 0.4 of a 'whole time equivalent' practice nurse.[29] Nurse-led PMS pilots tend to have a significantly 'richer' primary health care team, both in terms of the doctor–nurse ratio and the total clinical resource. However, it should be noted that the population served by the nine nurse-led pilots may be significantly different to the average, and many are associated with significant deprivation and high health needs.

Box 2.1

A day in the life of Teresa Kearney, Nurse Practitioner

PMS nurse-led pilot for travellers and homeless families

Acorns Surgery, Grays, Essex

'Manning the surgery begins at 10 a.m., which is comparatively late but, for us, appropriate given our client group. This enables me to sort out post, answer telephone queries or to be able to fit in a meeting before surgery commences. There is currently a great deal of interest in the PMS model and I handle a good few enquiries by telephone from PCTs, mostly those that are about to go live (for PMS) on 1 April 2001.

Surgery, however, inevitably overruns, finishing between 1–2 hours behind schedule. This is largely due to patients presenting with multiple and complex needs. The fact that the patient population is transient motivates both myself and my GP colleague to cover as much as possible in one consultation. This would be anathema to most primary care providers, with patient consultation times allocated to them at 5 to 7 minute intervals.

For us, a consultation may last 50 minutes, especially if an interpreter is present. When surgery eventually finishes, it's back to sorting out other presenting problems or queries that have arisen from various quarters, for example the trust or the PCG.

Lunch is usually eaten on the move or I miss it altogether; today it is while I travel to the local acute hospital. There I run a TB clinic in conjunction with one of the consultant chest physicians. This is a bi-monthly arrangement. I thought that it could improve the primary–secondary interface and at the same time raise the profile of the practice among secondary care colleagues. Another plus was the desire to provide continuity of care, as some patients would be referred to the acute hospital for screening. This has worked quite well, and those of my patients who do attend the clinic are both pleased and surprised to see a familiar face.

After this, I am off to a teenage strategy meeting. The last job of the day is to telephone the surgery to collect my messages and then I can look forward to home and the family.'

Table 2.1: Characteristics of the first wave nurse-led PMS pilots

Pilot	Main Characteristics	Go Live Date	Service Provider/Contract Holder	PMS Plus Services (if any)	Pilot Aims	List Size (1/12/00)	Staffing
Acorns	Services to travellers, homeless and refugees in Thurrock. Offers outreach services. Many non-English - speaking patients.	Oct 1998	South Essex Mental Health and Community NHS Trust	PMS Plus (Plus includes: – midwifery – child development)	Target vulnerable patient groups. Re-design services to be more patient focused. Maximise competencies of nurses and doctors.	1000	NP (1 WTE) GP (0.8 WTE)
Appleton Primary Care	New practice in affluent part of Warrington. Focus on use of IT and patient partnership.	Aug 1999	Warrington Community NHS Trust	PMS Plus: Community nursing services	Offer holistic and patient-focused services. Break down professional barriers. Offer 'good value'.	1000	NP (1 WTE) GP (1 WTE) PN (1 WTE)
Arch Day Centre	Branch surgery of existing GMS practice offering services to homeless people in Stoke.	Apr 1998	PMS GP	PMS only	Develop services for vulnerable young people. Increase access and provide user-friendly environment. Client participation. Partnership and collaboration with statutory and voluntary sector groups.	350 + 50 temp resident	NP (1 WTE) GP (as required) Substance misuse clinician\n\nGP input provided by linked PMS practice
Daruzzaman Care Centre	Replacement of existing GMS practice in Salford on death of GP.	Apr 1998	Independent nurse contractor	PMS Plus: Community nursing services	Offer patient-focused care. Emphasis on community/social priorities. Value, access, flexibility, choice and empowerment.	1950	NP (1 WTE) GP (2 WTE) – covering clinical, audit, training and research duties HV/DN
Edith Cavell Practice	New practice offering services to vulnerable groups (refugees, homeless, mentally ill, substance abusers). Now also providing wave 2 pilot.	Oct 1998	Community Health South London NHS Trust	PMS only	Improving access and services for vulnerable groups. Higher quality via structured approach to care. Close working with community groups. Develop links with RCN institute.	2600 (W1 pilot)	NP lead (1 WTE) GP (1.5 WTE)
Meadowfields Practice	New practice in Derby.	Aug 1998	Independent nurse contractor	PMS only	Shift in power base from GPs to wider team. Patients to be seen by most appropriate clinician. Involvement of patients in service design.	2500	PN (lead) (1 WTE) GP (1.25 WTE) PN (0.8 WTE)

Practice	Description	Date	Provider	Contract	Aims	List	Staffing
Morley Street Surgery	New practice in Brighton providing services to homeless people, including outreach services. Working in partnership with a range of voluntary and statutory agencies.	Oct 1998	South Downs Health Trust	PMS only	Target vulnerable patients. Enhanced NP role. Team-based approach with wider range of expertise within the team.	847	NP (1 WTE) GP (1.3 WTE)
The Spitalfields PMS Practice	PMS branch of a GMS practice providing services to homeless people in East London and the City.	Dec 1999	The Spitalfields Practice (GMS)	PMS	Target homeless populations: – street homeless – hostel homeless	500	NP (2 WTE) GP (1 WTE)
Valley Park Surgery	New surgery offering services to under-doctored area.	Nov 1998	Croydon and Surrey Downs Community NHS Trust	PMS Plus: Community nursing services	Improved access. Emphasis on community development.	1000	NP/HV (0.8 WTE) PN (1 WTE) GP (0.4 WTE) GP input contracted from PCG

3. What are nurse-led services?

Nurse leads ascribe a complex set of values to the term 'nurse-led primary care'. In Chapter 1, the development of the advanced level nurse practitioner was discussed. Certainly, the use of advanced nursing skills forms part of the definition of 'nurse-led primary care' but by no means the whole of it.

The nurse leads themselves have developed a multi-factorial understanding of what 'nurse-led primary care' means in practice. Interestingly, only part of this definition relates to the clinical contribution of the nurse lead. Nurse 'leadership' is as much a philosophical, as it is a clinical, construct.

Two distinct components of 'nurse-led primary care' can be identified within the context of PMS pilots:

(a) Implementation of enhanced nursing roles

Nurse leads emphasised that their pilots provided an opportunity to carry out extended nursing roles. The most important extended role is that of the clinical assessment and treatment of patients undifferentiated by need. The nurse leads described themselves as 'gate-keepers' and 'navigators' (terms usually ascribed within the NHS to the role of the GP). Therefore, this traditional GP role is being undertaken by (or at least shared with) nurses within the nine pilot sites.

> *Patients go to the GP because they don't know where else to go and I put myself in the place of the first port of call so that I can maybe navigate or help that person. If it's me, that's fine; if it's the GP, that's fine. But it may be [the] marriage guidance [service].*

Yet, while this role may be relatively unusual for nurses within primary care is it actually serving to 'extend' nursing roles into the domain of medicine? One nurse lead argued that the pilot was simply redressing an historical trend that had seen nursing roles eroded:

> *Doctors have actually taken on nursing roles and we are reclaiming nursing territory. Over the years, ordinary life has become medicalised.*

The nursing role of initial patient assessment (or 'triage') was also a hallmark of nurse-led care. However, this was carried out differently across the nine pilots. In some pilots, all urgent, same-day patient appointments are taken by the nurse lead. In others, patients may choose whether to see a nurse or a GP. For follow-up care, pilots are again organised differently and their patients experience different degrees of choice over which clinician they will see. One pilot was clear that it was always the patient's choice that they consulted. Another pilot describes a system of 'assisted decision-making':

> *For same day appointments, **we** [the nurses] make a decision ... every call is triaged by a nurse. ... But following that the nurse might make a decision [that the patient] needs to go into a GP ... The reason being we want to try to make the best use of clinician time and the best use of the patients' time.*

However, the existence of a nurse-led system of 'triage' within a primary care team is not, in itself, sufficient to define 'nurse-led primary care'. Many nurse practitioners within the NHS already carry out this role and have done so for a long time. Indeed, the third wave of PMS pilots that will 'go live' in April and October 2001 looks set to increase substantially the numbers of nurse practitioners within primary care. Yet the majority of these will work within a 'traditional' model of general practice and will not claim the title 'nurse-led'. Therefore, a further attribute is required to understand the meaning that nurse leads ascribe to 'nurse-led primary care'. This attribute is related to a specific value system that is promulgated within the primary care team.

(b) A 'nurse-led' value system

Nurse leads all emphasised that their pilots were based on an overt value system that renegotiated two sets of relationships: those between clinicians within the primary health care team and those between the team and their patients.

The relations between team members (particularly between nurses and doctors) are intended to reflect new values of equality and respect for complementary professional competencies. In part, this is intended to free nurses to use their skills to the full and to redress a power imbalance between doctors and nurses, allowing the latter to enjoy the autonomy so long enjoyed by the former:

> *The autonomy bit is really important too. It is not about carrying out a task because the GP says.*

> *It is about challenging how we have traditionally delivered the care, and that has always been medically led ... it's about the acknowledgement that nurses can do that.*

This desire to challenge the perceived *status quo* emerged from strongly held perceptions among the nurse leads that the professional culture of nurses was less conservative and more willing to promote patients' interests than that of traditional general practice:

> *If you were to say to doctors, 'Provide an open access service', it would terrify them, absolutely. Whereas, all the nurses you say that to say, 'Oh yeah, that's a really good idea.'*

Nurse leads also emphasised the importance of the non-profit-making nature of their pilots. This they contrasted to the incentives that existed for GPs under the general medical services contract:

> *[Nurse-led primary care] wants to put patients first; put service first rather than profit.*

> *[GMS] motivates [GPs] in a different way and then they get this mindset of saying: 'I've got to do that; I have got to reach that target because I have to be paid.'*

However, it is interesting to note that two of the nurse leads are independent contractors and not salaried employees. They might, in theory, be expected to be subject to the same incentives to 'profit maximise' as GPs (albeit without the same contractual target and fee-for-service incentives). That they have not suggests that contractual and organisational form alone is insufficient to determine the prevailing philosophy within a primary care organisation. Indeed, nurse leads explicitly recognised that many 'traditional' GMS practices pursued the same or similar philosophies as that expounded by nurse-led pilots. As one nurse lead suggested:

> *It's about philosophy, it's not about contract.*

This philosophy was underpinned by a belief that they had established a significantly different relationship with their patients. This reflected a mission to empower patients and to locate the work of the practices within the wider community inhabited by patients, taking account of their social concerns. Nurse leads emphasised their willingness to offer patients choice and responsibility in relation to their care. While nurse leads accepted that a minority of GMS practices aspired to a similar vision, nevertheless, they associated patient empowerment and interprofessional equality with nursing, rather than medical, values and culture. Doctors who concurred with this view were described, by one lead, as 'closet nurses'.

In many respects, therefore, the defining characteristic of the nurse-led pilots is not concerned with 'leadership' by nurses at all, but by an equality of opportunity, mutual respect among team members and a focus on the needs of patients. In these circumstances, the title 'nurse-led' may be misleading, something recognised by the nurse leads themselves:

> *'Nurse-led' ... was a tag that got used politically to say that we weren't 'doctor-led'.*

What we are saying is there is a different way to deliver primary care that may be led by anybody.

Box 3.2: Daruzzaman Care Centre

'Commissioning for Well-being'

The Daruzzaman Care Centre pilot in Salford is one of three projects in Manchester and Salford to develop a new arrangement to involve the community in the work and governance of statutory agencies. Adapting the school governor model, the pilot has created a governing body comprising:

10 patients

2 city councillors

1 PCG member

2 staff members from the pilot

The governing body has been delegated the control of the PMS budget (together with some resources from the PCG and local authority Community Committee) and will work with the team to develop more patient-centred services on behalf of the wider community. The age range of governors is from 16 to 65 years.

In this respect, 'leadership' by nurses, within an environment for so long dominated by doctors, has important symbolic value, even if it may not accurately reflect the operation of the primary health care team. In order that nurses may operate within a professionally equitable environment, it appears necessary to ascribe a formal leadership role, even if that role is not adopted or maintained in the long term:

Whether I'm a nurse or a doctor or whatever, I really don't give a monkey's anymore. I think it's all about patient focus and I'm a carer, a person who provides care. And whether that's with a nursing background or not, it's not that important to me. But I appreciate it is important to the [nursing] profession.

However, some nurse leads felt that professional equality within the team was an aspiration rather than a current reality. To reach the desired state of equality, it was first necessary for a nurse formally to be seen to be in a position of authority within the team. During this time, at least two nurse leads felt that the burden of leadership was tangible:

> *That nurse-led element is very real because what that actually is telling me is that I'm responsible for all of that other stuff [e.g. managing the practice] and what my GP would do is ... come in and he would just do his clinical work and go home.*

> *I went into it very enthusiastic and excited and I put a lot into it and I made myself ill in the end. I was working 60 hours a week trying to hold it all together.*

PMS – reaching the parts not reached by GMS

Perhaps not surprisingly, given their philosophical underpinning, the nurse-led pilots are strongly associated with vulnerable, or traditionally under-served, populations. Seven of the nine pilots were established in response to the needs of particular types of patients (such as the homeless and refugees) or to serve areas with generally inadequate access to primary care services.

This association between PMS pilots and deprivation or particular patient needs has been remarked upon before[30,31] and features among the governmental aims set out for PMS.[32] Therefore, this aspect of the nurse-led pilots stems from their inclusion within the PMS movement in general, rather than as a feature of their nurse-led orientation. However, it is notable that a far greater proportion of nurse-led pilots are seeking to fill the gaps left by GMS than is true for PMS pilots as a whole. Are nurse-led services particularly suited to this type of work? Nurse leads feel that they are. In particular, they suggest that nursing culture and skills appear well-suited to working within complex social–clinical environments and in promoting wider public health within communities (although many primary care doctors might well claim the same thing).

Nurse leads contrast starkly their new model of care with that of 'traditional' general practice:

> *We did manage to work in a different way ... which was very different to anything ... I've done before; going out into the community and finding [out what] people needed and ... getting feedback from them rather than just providing a service that we thought was appropriate.*

> *[In my previous GMS practice] there was no continuity of care. There was no one actually saying or highlighting a need; they were just being 'sticky-plastered'.*

One consequence of the emergence of these new types of pilot appears to be a growing division between services for vulnerable populations and mainstream primary care. Nurse-led pilots have a tendency to act as beacons for particular patient groups, drawing them away from other practices. Nurse leads were aware that neighbouring practices may also deliberately direct certain of their own registered patients (or people seeking to register) towards the new service:

> *Our local GPs now would say [to patients] ... 'Go to that practice', and that's fine because in many respects they would get a better deal from us anyway because we are tailored and hopefully more responsive to their need than the other practice populations in the locality.*

While the advantage to patients who register with practices that are willing and able to care for them is self-evident, it raises an uncomfortable issue of restricted patient choice. If other general practices in the area feel able to divest themselves of responsibilities towards certain population groups, these patients may effectively have a choice of only one source of primary care. Similarly, the spectre of general practices 'picking and choosing' patients sits uneasily with the vision of a comprehensive health service offering equal access to all. As one nurse lead suggested:

PMS is seen as the sponge that absorbs the difficulties, whereas good GMS should be doing this anyway.

4. Pushing back the professional boundaries?

As has already been discussed, government health policy relies on the successful development of new and extended roles for nurses. Nurse-led PMS pilots represent an obvious vanguard for this movement in primary care and a 'trial run' for this policy.

Significantly, nurse leads expressed serious reservations about the way in which extended nursing roles in primary care had been introduced and the feasibility for their wider promulgation within the NHS. Of particular concern was the rise in the popularity of the nurse practitioner role (or, at least, the use of that title) and the relative lack of regulation and quality control over the practice of these nurses. Many new nurse practitioner roles are being generated through walk-in centres and in 'standard' (i.e. not 'nurse-led') PMS pilot proposals. Nurse leads drew attention to the fact that no nationally agreed competencies, standards or training curricula exist for the role of 'nurse practitioner'.

> *People have done a three-day course or a six-day course or a six-week course and call themselves [a nurse practitioner]. There is no underpinning for it; there is no basic standard and we need to have that laid down, so that nationally there is the same standard applied ... We [nurse leads] are all nurse practitioners; we are supposed to be leading on the cutting edge of primary care and we have not got any legitimate standards.*

In the experience of some nurse leads, many applicants for nurse practitioner posts do not have appropriate experience to carry out the role safely:

> *Certainly, interviewing for the walk-in centre, they still have nurses that think that they can just come straight out [of hospital] and work in the community, and they can't.*

While clinical governance processes at local level are intended to provide a quality assurance framework for the work of the nurse-led pilots, the experience of the nurse leads suggests that this is, so far, ineffective:

> *You end up with a clinical governance lead who says ... 'Well, we won't bother coming to you because you are so far above the rest we have to concentrate on those who aren't.' ... So nobody is doing any clinical governance with us; we haven't had a visit.*

> *[Clinical governance leads] are just not necessarily looking at our competency and what we are doing.*

Nurse leads identify the development of explicit standards for nurse practitioners as an urgent priority and are critical of the United Kingdom Central Council in their management of the emergence of advanced nursing roles in primary care to date:

> *[The UKCC is] failing because they are not protecting my patients from me ... They should have been through the front door on a virtually monthly basis saying, 'Are these people safe?' ... Just because I have a high profile they assume I'm safe.*

> *The issue is all about competency ... so what we actually have to develop is the competencies necessary to practice at the advanced level.*

Nurse leads recognised that their position as 'pioneers' of new nursing roles made them a potent symbol for nurses elsewhere. As one nurse lead suggested: 'There was a pressure that the whole of the nursing profession were looking to me to make it a success.' However, they were concerned that the next cadre of nurse leads was not materialising. Instead, a vacuum was forming:

> *I don't feel the nurses are behind [us], champing at the bit to follow.*

If I left tomorrow, then I could name six nurses in the whole country prepared to take my job.

There is a trickle [of potential nurse leads] and I don't know if that trickle will grow.

In part, they ascribed this reticence among nurses to step into nurse-led roles as a response to the difficulties the nine pilots had faced in establishing their pilots:

Maybe there are motivated people out there but ... I wouldn't want anybody to face what I had to face because I don't think it is fair.

These difficulties with implementation are discussed in more depth below.

Interprofessional relations

In the previous chapter, the nurse leads' vision of interprofessional equality and co-operation was described. This was at the very centre of their aims for their pilots. To what extent has this vision found its expression in reality?

In many pilots, the internal team dynamics were consistent with the vision. However, in a minority of pilots some issues of power emerged between doctors and nurses within the pilots. At its most benign, this manifested itself through GP control of the management of patient care, in particular retaining the power of deciding which clinician would see which patient:

There is a small minority [of patient care] that is GP controlled. By [the GP] looking [at the appointment list] ... and saying, 'I'm sure they are going to come in with that, I'd better see them' ... that is still very GP controlled.

The existing legal framework (particularly that patients can only be registered with a doctor, that a doctor must be present whenever patients were treated and the current requirement that GPs must sign virtually all prescriptions) has undermined the nurses' ability to manage the pilots independently. Where relationships between medical and nursing team members were good and where they shared a common vision of practice, this problem had been overcome. In most pilots, doctors and nurse leads worked hard together to implement flexible systems. However, in one pilot significant problems emerged within the team over the interpretation of 'nurse-led' services and over the respective roles of doctors and nurses within the pilot:

Although it was supposed to be nurse led, the power was still all in the hands of the doctors; so nothing changed really ... if the doctor chose to, they could actually use that power, which was very frustrating.

So in terms of professions working more closely together, actually we were doctors and nurses at war in the end; worse than in any other job I'd been in.

This pilot saw the rapid departure of two nurse leads within two years of its inception.

While good interprofessional relations could generally be maintained within pilots, nurse leads experienced a significant degree of suspicion, and sometimes hostility, from neighbouring GPs and local medical committees (LMCs). One focus of this hostility was the employment of salaried GPs. Nurse leads perceived the concerns of local doctors (particularly LMCs) to stem mainly from concerns that salaried general practice would undermine the system of GMS and represented the 'thin end of the wedge'. This has been reported elsewhere[33] and appears to be an issue related to PMS pilots generally, rather than nurse-led pilots specifically.

However, some scepticism by local doctors with the actual model of nurse-led care was reported. This may well have heightened the local hostility felt towards the pilots. Nurse leads felt that they were caricatured as 'oddball' or 'bizarre'. Some pilots found themselves penalised by local decisions to refuse them membership of the out-of-hours co-operative or to overcharge for membership. One pilot was charged £21,000 for annual membership of the co-operative, instead of the £7000 that they had expected to pay.

Nurse leads questioned whether interprofessional tension was heightened if nurse-led pilots sought to provide mainstream services, rather than a service aimed at vulnerable groups poorly served by GMS. A manager of one nurse-led pilot serving vulnerable populations described the reaction of local GPs when plans were advanced for a second wave nurse-led pilot serving a more general population:

> *We set-up the nurse-led PMS pilot for homeless, travellers and refugees and [the view of local doctors was] ... 'Oh yeah, nurses can do it and we can get on with the big boy's stuff.' When we tried to get a PMS pilot for the ordinary population, we were stopped by the medics ... all of a sudden we were encroaching on what was traditionally their territory ... to say I got assassinated by the medical colleagues ... was an understatement ... The bottom line was also that they would be losing income ... [Patients] were also frightened because their GPs were telling them ... 'If you join that practice you will never be able to come back to mine.'*

However, notwithstanding these early difficulties, nurse leads also reported that the sense of hostility and isolation that they felt diminished as the number of PMS pilots increased nationally. Again, this is consistent with other evaluation findings that suggest that, over time, tensions between pilots and primary care colleagues have dissipated.[34]

The primary–secondary care interface

If the Government's strategy to re-engineer the primary health care team is to succeed, the interface between primary and secondary care also requires renegotiation. A key attribute for nurse-led primary care is that nurses can directly access diagnostic services and make and receive referrals from the hospital sector. This is set out as one of the Chief Nursing Officer's ten challenges for nurses.

The experience of nurse leads in implementing this has been varied. While some hospitals have responded quickly to the changes imposed upon them by primary care, others have proved more inflexible. This may not be wholly surprising. The nurse-led pilots are few in number and hospitals may not have been automatically aware of their presence or their objectives (although, other primary care nurses in GMS or in 'standard' PMS pilots, no doubt, will also have attempted to introduce similar changes).

Table 4.1: Clinical relationships with hospital services

Pilot	Acorns	Appleton Primary Care	Arch Day Centre	Daruzza-man Care Centre	Edith Cavell Practice	Meadow-fields Practice	Morley Street Surgery	The Spital-fields PMS Practice	Valley Park Surgery
Nature of Arrange-ment	Informal	Formal	Informal	Formal	Informal	Informal	Informal	Not yet estab.	Informal
Acceptance of referrals	Most specialties	Most specialties	A range of specialties	All specialties	A range of specialties	All specialties	Most specialties	N/A	Some specialties
Consultant letters	Letters to GP	Some letters to nurse	Some letters to nurse	Letters to team	Letters to nurse	Some letters to nurse	Some letters to nurse	N/A	Some letters back to nurse

Table 4.1 shows the degree of variability between the nurse leads in terms of making referrals to hospital consultants (and having those referrals accepted) and in receiving letters back from consultants or diagnostic departments. Only two pilots have negotiated formal arrangements with hospital NHS trusts. The majority rely on informal arrangements agreed with individual hospital clinicians and departments. These arrangements have evolved and, over time, led to a gradual extension of the range of specialties prepared to accept referrals from nurse leads. However, few nurse leads can expect a standard response from their hospital providers and may have to undertake substantial work to develop relationships that support the philosophy of their pilot.

Few nurse leads have referrals accepted by all specialties without exception. However, in many cases, even informal systems function quite well. The extent to which some hospitals have radically reviewed the nature of their clinical relationships with primary care nurses should not be underestimated. Many consultants have undertaken a significant culture change:

> *Any referral I send comes back to me personally and I have a relationship with the consultants which two years ago, they say, there is no way [they] would have got into.*

> *[My relationship with the hospital] was excellent ... I never had a referral refused and I was getting letters back to me ... I have to confess that when I was doing acute referrals ... I never actually said, 'I'm a nurse practitioner', but I always put that on my letters. That was cheating in a way, I know.*

> *I haven't actually had [referrals] sent back to me, but there is some degree of opposition in the acute unit. I've been bashing on the acute [hospital] front doors since I started and its starting to change.*

Where problems existed, they were likely to reflect distrust, by particular hospital staff, of the competency of nurse leads to deal appropriately with clinical information. This has caused significant disruption at practice level and has served to undermine the aims and operation of the pilots. The response of hospital staff can be idiosyncratic:

> *Every X-ray now gets phoned up to see if the doctors saw it or the nurse ... some of the labs are OK, but not ultrasound. The same applies to microbiology. It has caused a huge problem because all they keep doing is sending stuff back saying, 'Doctor unknown' ... I am admitting what I'm doing – 'This is a nurse-led PMS pilot' – and it is causing massive, massive problems.*

> *I'm not allowed ultrasound scans although I have the occasional one. I can get an MRI scan.*

Nurse leads, however, have noted an improvement in their ability to refer to (and receive information from) their local hospitals. In one case, the reticence of consultants to receive nurse practitioner referrals did not extend to their private medical practice:

> *Where I'm working is affluent ... and I've got all these people in BUPA. So all these ... consultants who have been refusing to accept*

my referrals for years, I now write to them as BUPA and I'm getting,
'Dear [name]' letters back.

Yet, despite their problems, nurse leads do not necessarily interpret consultant behaviour as simple professional intransigence. They have considerable sympathy with what they see as a professional dilemma for consultants. This stems from their concerns about the lack of recognised standards and competencies that underpin the role of nurse practitioner. Consultants, they argue, are not able to judge the validity of any referral that they receive from a nurse practitioner:

Our profession has never sorted out what is a proper standard of examination and diagnosis. And therefore the consultant cannot be sure that the history is correct, that the examination has not missed anything and it is unethical therefore to accept it.

The problem is that our house is not in order.

We bat [the consultants] into a corner. But it's difficult because we have identified the need but they cannot be sure of how that need is identified.

5. Implementing the pilots – 'swimming against the tide'

All nurse leads emphasised the struggles that they had undergone in implementing their pilots. Introducing a radical new model of service has not been easily achieved. Many of the obstacles they faced were bureaucratic; the automatic response of the NHS was to expect that the roles undertaken by the nurse leads would, instead, be carried out by doctors. Partner organisations have proved insufficiently flexible to adapt quickly to the new arrangements:

> *We are trying to change 50 years of history, but when you actually look at minimum data sets, all that it says is 'doctor'. The Department says 'doctor', all the software from the computers starts with 'doctor' and 'doctor number', and trying to change all that for just a few of us is really quite difficult.*

This inflexibility caused considerable stress among nurse leads and made their task even more difficult than they felt it needed to be:

> *One of the big difficulties that I have, and I'm sure all of my colleagues have, is that you actually haven't got the toolbox to do [your] job. And that is exceedingly difficult and very frustrating and causes a great deal of grief ... it is almost like trying to undertake a job with one hand tied behind your back and sometimes both.*

> *I was wading through treacle ... I can't get on and do things because I'm blocked.*

What lessons can future nurse-led pilots learn from the experience of the first wave? A number of issues relating to implementation emerge.

Regulatory obstacles

Nurse leads identified a range of regulatory obstacles that hindered them in fulfilling their roles. The signatures of primary care nurses are not acceptable to the Benefits Agency in relation to absence from work due to sickness, nor are they accepted on death certificates:

> *Somebody who is off sick, especially somebody who is off sick long term, is a prime example of somebody [for whom] nursing skills are absolutely good because you are in a better position to gain the whole social set – and likely to have more time to help people to address that issue as to why they can't work.*

In addition, patients can only be registered with a GP, irrespective of whether the pilot is nurse-led (or even that the doctor may be directly employed by the nurse).

Of perhaps greater significance is the highly restricted ability of nurses to prescribe pharmaceuticals. While the ability to prescribe is critical to their work, nurse leads all felt that their current scope (under the existing nurse prescribing scheme) was minimal and inadequate:

> *We can only prescribe cream and cotton wool.*

The pilots have been operational during the time that the Department of Health has been reviewing policy in relation to prescribing (particularly the prescribing rights of non-medical professionals). However, this debate will not be concluded within the three-year life span of the first wave pilots. Consequently, nurse-led pilots have developed informal arrangements with the GPs in their teams, whereby prescriptions are routinely signed having been drawn up by the nurse lead. This may or may not include a clinical review of the patient's notes by the GP prior to signing.

Nurse leads have been careful to prepare prescriptions only within their own competencies. Even so, any GP signing such a prescription is felt, in the words of one nurse lead, to be 'on the boundaries of legality'. This implies a considerable professional and personal risk for GPs within nurse-led pilots and one nurse lead suggested that GPs had 'put their neck on the line'. Such an arrangement between nurse leads and GPs is *de facto* creating full rights for nurse prescribing. It is clear that policy development 'on the ground' has moved in advance of the official policy framework being developed by the Department of Health.

Project sponsors and local champions

As has been noted, five of the nine pilots are sponsored and managed by community NHS trusts. Many of these trusts established the schemes out of a desire to push back professional boundaries and to offer services to previously under-served populations. Notwithstanding their motivations, nurse leads identified significant disadvantages associated with community trust-managed schemes.

In particular, nurse leads identified a lack of autonomy over the management of their pilot and felt themselves the victims of an excessive bureaucracy. Community trusts were perceived as generally ignorant about the operational detail of general practice, nor could they respond rapidly to the day-to-day needs of primary care organisation. As public bodies, they had a considerable bureaucracy that could not be sidestepped. Consequently, some nurse leads felt the presence of a dead weight that slowed down the achievement of their aims and even, at times, stopped them providing basic services:

> *[Community trusts] don't understand how primary care works. They don't understand how a practice operates. And yet they're right in the middle of primary care ... You know you go through various trials to try and get something done but they just don't appreciate it ... there is still this heavy bureaucratic nightmare to navigate before you can achieve your goal.*

> *It is embarrassing; we have so many red letters. We have been blacklisted by all sorts of suppliers ... because the trust doesn't pay the bills.*

Our fridge broke down and I was four weeks without a fridge because Electrolux wouldn't send me a new fridge because the trust had not paid for it and it took four weeks. Can you imagine a GP surgery anywhere else without a fridge? ... Had I been in my previous practice and managed by a GP ... he would've said, 'There's a cheque, go get a fridge.'

However, it cannot be inferred from this that the independent contractor or general practice model of pilot necessarily provides a more satisfactory vehicle. Independent contractor nurse leads commented that their position, while maximising autonomy, provided few, if any, mechanisms for their own personal support. The independent contractor model of nurse-led primary care can result in the nurse feeling isolated, often in the face of considerable resistance or hostility to the work that they are trying to undertake:

Nurses ring me and say, 'I want to be an independent practitioner', and I do my utmost to put them off ... because I don't think it is necessary. I don't think it is helpful to them as individuals and I don't think it is that helpful to the NHS ... [the problem] is the isolation.

Nurse leads identified that local champions were important in the success of any pilot. Within a trust-managed pilot, operational managers have been able to support and encourage nurse leads. This has been seen as a means to minimise stress on the nurse lead. However, it has not been forthcoming in all the trust-managed pilots and, where it has been absent, this has been to the detriment of the pilot:

You need political champions at health authority or trust level. You need people who are big hitters who actually are on board with what we are doing.

Everybody hasn't got [a manager] at a senior level to say, 'Get off their backs and let them do their work.'

A minority of trust-managed pilots also suggested that senior managers within community trusts may not offer the same degree of support as their colleagues closer to the pilot. In particular, two pilots expressed the view that senior medical clinicians within their trusts were 'anti-nurse' or, at best, indifferent to the nursing objectives of the pilot. This, again, suggests interprofessional tensions and a reluctance, on the part of doctors, to embrace a nurse-led model of primary care.

> *I think I get managerial support ... I think they recognise the role you are aiming to fulfil. But, because then my next line of support [within the trust] is medical, [the support] just goes.*

It appears, therefore, that nurse leads face a trade-off between autonomy and personal support. Trust-managed pilots may provide greater personal support to their nurse leads, but at the cost of an inadequate management support service. Independent contractor nurses are able to manage their own organisations, but must face any resistance to their pilot largely alone (although health authorities have, in some cases, provided support).

The issue of support is significant. Nurse leads clearly feel that they face a degree of exposure far greater than that experienced by other health professionals:

> *I had no idea of the big games that are being played out there ... the arena is not built for us to operate in.*

> *The nursing profession is being expected to push out the boundaries ... to a hugely greater extent than any GP would be expected to ... I can't think of any GPs that would actually put their position on the line.*

> *The PCG are now seeing me as a test tube ... Because if it works, then it's their idea, and if it doesn't then it's the weird nurse down the road.*

6. Conclusion

More than two years into their pilots, the nine nurse-led pilots have achieved a great deal. New practices have been formed, many thousands of patients are being served and nurses have been responsible for developing and leading teams of primary care professionals. In a very real sense, the nurse-led PMS pilots are putting in place the radical vision for health care called for by Tony Blair and his government.

And yet these developments have not been without personal costs for the nurses involved. A punishing workload and a highly politicised environment, with resistance or blockages from many quarters, appear to have been the norm. Certainly the NHS juggernaut will not turn on a sixpence. Nor should the 'forces of conservatism' be underestimated. Nurse leads have faced professional and bureaucratic obstacles that have proved quite unyielding. To the extent that the pilots have been successful, this has been despite the 'system' and not because of it. However, this is not to say that, having been the brainchild of ministers, the nine leads have been abandoned to their fates. As one nurse lead commented wryly: 'Never have nine nurses had such access to ministers.'

What can we learn from their experiences? First, that 'nurse-led' primary care (or at least this incarnation of it) is about more than changing professional roles. The nurse leads have aspired to create a service and a culture that has patient needs and interprofessional equality at its centre. This transcends any model of 'nurse leadership' and even PMS itself. This philosophy has always had its adherents within GMS; perhaps PMS makes it more easy to achieve.

Second, the model of enhanced nursing roles is not without controversy. Certainly, the medical jury is still out. Some nurses encountered resistance from within their own team or within the hierarchies of their NHS trusts. One nurse lead talked of doctors and nurses 'at war'. More commonly, suspicion emerged from other local doctors. Nurse leadership is but one further change heralded by PMS pilots that has, more generally, raised the hackles of a section of 'traditional' general practice.

Yet it would be wrong to overplay the resistance faced by the pilots. Perhaps surprisingly, pilots made good progress in winning referral rights within their local hospitals. However, this was not universal and remains mainly an informal arrangement, with some consultants feeling able to ignore the reality of the extended nursing role. These consultants still prefer to communicate only with other doctors.

Third, the provision of dedicated services for vulnerable population groups raises some interesting ethical issues. New PMS pilots have proved popular because they are sympathetic and skilled in dealing with particular patient groups. Yet, they also let neighbouring practices 'off the hook' in relation to these patients. GMS practices are perceived to direct refugees or homeless people to PMS practices, rather than accept them onto their own lists. Is this simply a sensible use of scarce skills or is it the creation of 'ghetto primary care'? Does this fly in the face of a vision of an equitable NHS with the disadvantaged offered nurse-led care while the rest receive GP-led services? Interestingly, most medical resistance to the nurse-led model occurred when nurses had the temerity to attempt to offer services to the 'mainstream' population. This perhaps suggests that interprofessional rivalry remains muted, only for as long as nurse-led services remain 'on the margins'.

Fourth, the issue of excessive bureaucracy was raised. In part, this relates to NHS and welfare regulations that do not recognise the new role of nurses in primary care. These regulations should be amended (in the case of nurse prescribing, a liberalisation of the current legal framework is imminent). More worrying, perhaps, was the bureaucracy associated with NHS trust management of PMS pilots. Nurse leads were poorly supported by their trusts in many cases. Community NHS trusts were also perceived to know little about primary care and certainly failed to provide the responsive management support required within a general practice setting. As these trusts are transformed into primary care trusts (PCTs), what does this tell us about the future for PCT-led PMS pilots?

PCTs, with primary care at their heart, might be expected to have a greater degree of knowledge of (and perhaps sympathy for) the day-to-day needs of PMS practices, whether nurse led or not. Whether they will be able to overcome the tendency to bureaucratic inertia, so common in large organisations, is another matter. With similar public accountability frameworks to other bodies, PCTs may not be any quicker to purchase the new practice refrigerator. Will PCTs be sympathetic to the aims of nurse-led pilots? Again, it is too early to say. PCTs may certainly share the vision of needs-led services, but will they want to challenge the power balance between GPs and nurses? Community trusts contain powerful nursing hierarchies and may be expected to support nurse-led schemes. PCTs, in contrast, have seen the relative importance of community nursing issues diluted.

Lastly, and perhaps most important of all, do we have the right infrastructure to take forward a new model of primary care nursing? Nurse leads had significant concerns about the free use of the term 'nurse practitioner' and cast doubt on the training and competencies that currently underpin that role. As leading nurse practitioners themselves, this message should give pause for thought. Nurse leads raised the spectre of inadequate quality control and monitoring, both locally at practice level and nationally by professional bodies. Certainly, they appeared to receive little external professional support as they developed new and personally demanding roles. If the Chief Nursing Officer's vision of extended nursing roles is to be realised, these are issues requiring urgent resolution. The transformation of the UKCC and National Boards into the new Nursing and Midwifery Council should provide a useful stimulus for a wider debate on leadership, quality assurance and role development in nursing.

So what can we deduce about the Government's strategy to increase the contribution of nurses as part of a new approach to 'demand management'? Certainly there is now a welter of evidence which supports the view that nurses are able successfully to carry out extended clinical roles at acceptable cost and with high patient satisfaction. The gradually emerging evidence base in relation to PMS pilots suggests that they provide a good vehicle for allowing nurses to innovate and to carry out new roles. Other evaluations of nurse-led PMS pilots suggest that patients and practice staff are willing and able to embrace this new model with enthusiasm (although evidence about the cost-effectiveness of this model is, so far, not available).

This evaluation has sought to understand the experiences of a group of pioneers as they have sought to implement an ambitious personal and professional agenda. It has identified some problems that need to be addressed if widespread implementation of nurse-led care is to be effective. These problems, while significant, are not insurmountable and, in the case of extended nurse prescribing, the solution may already be in hand. Perhaps the most challenging issue is to address the cultural divide between doctors and nurses. The cultural dissonance between the two professions, highlighted in other work and discussed in Chapter 1, has been confirmed. Nurse leads see their own professional culture as more patient-oriented than that of doctors. Whether doctors would recognise this diagnosis is a rather different question. However, what is important is that nurses perceive a cultural divide to exist. This must be addressed if the trust and teamwork necessary for the Government's radical new vision is to be achieved.

If we can tentatively conclude that nurse-led pilots have begun to deliver a new model of care, however, a further question is raised – are the nurses necessary for the Government's 'new NHS' out there? Nurse leads doubted that they were. Clearly, both the medical and nursing professions are facing a crisis in recruitment. However, the perceived lack of successors to the first wave of nurse leads may also be a reflection of the difficulties experienced by the pioneers. As one lead commented:

> *I'm not sure I would advise anyone to do it really, sadly. At this stage I think there is a lot more things that would need to change before it can be successful.*

Nurse leads may prove to be a vanguard without an army.

References

[1] Jenkins C. Personal medical services – new opportunities. In: Lewis R, Gillam S, eds. *Transforming primary care: personal medical services in the new NHS.* London: King's Fund, 1999: 18–28.

[2] Walsh N, Andre C, Barnes M, Huntington J, Rogers H, Baines D. *New opportunities for primary care? A second year report of first wave PMS pilots in England.* Project Report No. 14. Birmingham: HSMC, 2000.

[3] Blair T. Speech to House of Commons. 22 March 2000.

[4] Milburn A. Speech to Annual Congress of the Royal College of Nurses. 5 April 2000.

[5] Secretary of State for Health. *The NHS Plan: a plan for investment, a plan for reform.* Cm 4818-I. London: The Stationery Office, 2000.

[6] Department of Health. *Statistical bulletin – statistics for general medical practitioners in England: 1989–1999.* London: Department of Health, 2000.

[7] Royal College of Nursing. *Nurse practitioners in primary health care – role definition.* London: Royal College of Nursing, 1989.

[8] Shum C, Humphreys A, Wheeler D, Cochrane M, Skoda S, Clement, S. Nurse management of patients with minor illnesses in general practice: multicentre, randomised controlled trial. *BMJ* 2000; 320: 1038–43.

[9] Kinnersley P, Anderson E, Parry K, Clement J, Archard L, Turton P, Stainthorpe A, Fraser A, Butler C C, Rogers C. Randomised controlled trial of nurse practitioner versus general practitioner care for patients requesting 'same day' consultations in primary care. *BMJ* 2000; 320: 1043–48.

[10] Venning P, Durie A, Roland M, Roberts C, Leese B. Randomised controlled trial comparing cost-effectiveness of general practitioners and nurse practitioners in primary care. *BMJ* 2000; 320: 1048–53.

[11] Mundinger M O, Kane R L, Lenz E R, Totten A M, Tsai W Y, Cleary P D, Friedewald W T, Siu A L, Shelanski M L. Primary care outcomes in patients treated by nurse practitioners or physicians. *JAMA* 2000; 283 (1): 59–68.

[12] Lister G, Cutler P, Dado K, Summerell N, Reilly C, Fletcher J. *Nurse practitioner evaluation project: final report.* Uxbridge: Coopers and Lybrand, 1996.

[13] NHS Executive. *Nurse prescribing: implementing the scheme across England.* HSC 1998/232. London: NHS Executive, 1998.

[14] Department of Health. *Patient group directions (England only).* HSC 2000/026. London: The Stationery Office, 2000.

[15] Department of Health. *Consultation on proposals to extend nurse prescribing.* London: The Stationery Office, 2000.

[16] Elston S, Holloway I. The impact of recent primary care reforms in the UK on interprofessional working in primary care centres. *Journal of Interprofessional Care* 2001; 15 (1): 19–27.

[17] Dingwall R, McIntosh J. Teamwork in theory and practice. In: Dingwall R, McIntosh J, eds. *Readings in the sociology of nursing.* Edinburgh: Churchill Livingstone, 1978: 118–34.

[18] Salvage J, Smith R. Doctors and nurses: doing it differently. *BMJ* 2000; 320: 1019–20.

[19] National Primary Care Research and Development Centre. *Cultural differences between medicine and nursing: implications for primary care.* Manchester: NPCRDC, University of Manchester, 1997.

[20] Gardner L. Nurse-led Primary Care Act pilot schemes: threat or opportunity? *Nursing Times* 1998; 94 (27): 52–53.

[21] Chapple A, Sergison M. Challenging tradition. *Nursing Times* 1999; 95 (12): 32–33.

[22] Walsh N, Huntington J. Testing the pilots. *Nursing Times* 2000; 96 (33): 32–33.

[23] Walsh N, André C, Barnes M, Huntington J, Rogers H, Baines D. *New opportunities for primary care? A second year report of first wave PMS pilots in England.* Birmingham: HSMC, 2000.

[24] Chapple A, Rogers A, Macdonald W, Sergison M. Patients' perceptions of changing professional boundaries and the future of 'nurse-led' services. *Primary Health Care Research and Development* 2000; 1: 51–59.

[25] Lewis R, Gillam S, eds. *Transforming primary care: personal medical services in the new NHS.* London: King's Fund, 1999.

[26] National Primary Care Research and Development Centre. *Cultural differences between medicine and nursing: implications for primary care.* Manchester: NPCRDC, University of Manchester, 1997.

[27] Jones D. Nurse-led pilots. In: Lewis R, Gillam S, eds. *Transforming primary care: personal medical services in the new NHS.* London, King's Fund, 1999: 41–50.

[28] Mudinger M O, Kane R L, Lenz E R, Totten A M, Tsai W Y, Cleary P D, Friedewald W T, Siu A L, Shelanski M L. Primary care outcomes in patients treated by nurse practitioners or physicians. *JAMA* 2000; 283 (1): 59–68.

[29] Department of Health. *Statistical bulletin – statistics for general medical practitioners in England: 1989–1999.* Leeds: Department of Health, 2000.

[30] Jenkins C, Lewis R. Reducing inequality. In: Lewis R, Gillam S, eds. *Transforming primary care: personal medical services in the new NHS.* London: King's Fund, 1999: 29–40.

[31] Carter Y, Curtis S, Harding G, Maguire A, Meads G, Riley A, Ross P, Underwood M. Addressing inequalities. In: *National evaluation of first wave NHS personal medical services pilots: integrated interim report from four research projects.* Manchester: NPCRDC, 2000: 13–15.

[32] NHS Executive. *Personal medical services: application process for third wave pilots.* HSC 2000/018. Leeds: NHS Executive, 2000.

[33] Lewis R, Jenkins C, Gillam S. *Personal medical services pilots in London – rewriting the red book.* London: King's Fund, 1999.

[34] Walsh N, Allen L, Baines D, Barnes M. *Taking off: a first year report of the personal medical services (PMS) pilots in England.* Birmingham: HSMC, 1999.